LET'S TALK ABOUT END OF LIFE PSYCHOTHERAPY

BIDO AGUESSY

Table of Contents

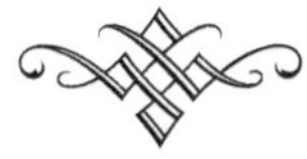

Introduction

At the *end of life*, Pastoral Care, Psychology, and Psychiatry converge. The End of Life can be compared to a person dropped at a train station, with a one-way ticket to a still unknown destination. While at the train station, the anxiety due to fear of the unknown–of the new destination, the station's discomfort, and the family's concern become the main causes of a person's emotional and psychological trauma. Though psychiatry and psychology can address the unbalanced chemical problem and some of the root causes of the anxiety, they both need a metaphysical approach to address the hope of the prospect of a new destination. Of course, the new destination in the case of the elderly in the long-term care facility is a possible life after death. This intervention will be theological, which is mostly called pastoral or spiritual care.

The limit of psychiatry and psychology at the end

of life is obvious but not acknowledged. This became a fact during the pandemic of Covid 19. Many residents were passing, visits were restricted, and the medical community had limited answers to people. Spiritual care was on-demand, even with people who'd earlier had little use for it. Any psychological intervention was theologically based on giving hope to a patient troubled by the fear of the unknown. The presence of a chaplain was enough to bring comfort to the staff, family members, and patients.

Before we continue our adventure with the *end of life*, let's stop at a long term care facility and spend time with some residents.

I

Time in a long-term care facility

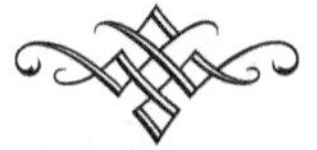

Walking through the Valley of
the Shadow of Death

Today Mrs. Green is admitted to hospice. At 75 years of age, her cancer is now out of control, and after a long period of hesitation, she finally accepted the palliative care approach. Mrs. Green is not religious but considers herself spiritual. She has been living in a long-term care facility for the last three years. Her depression started when her house was sold, and her new life began in another setting. That depression became complicated when she was admitted to hospice. Torn between acceptance and the fear of the unknown, her mood is now sinusoidal (waving up and down.) Spiritual and believing in God, she's wondered why God hasn't called her sooner.

On the other hand, she fears the unknown world

that she is going to. In this long-term care facility, she has many friends, and sometimes, she will see that they are missing, and the silence is loud. (Of course, they have gone to be with the Lord.) She is conscious of it and awaiting her turn. She loves bingo, the most interesting event everyone seems to look forward to daily. As she faces her mortality, Mrs. Green is suffering from late-life depression, a complicated depressive state. She tried to prepare for it, but it seems that there is no formula for this.

Across the hallway is Mrs. Red. She is in her late 80s and has lived in the facility for the last five years. Mrs. Red is extremely disciplined. This causes a clash between her and the staff. Mrs. Red always wants to know the name of her nurse, her aide. She likes things to be done with promptitude. After supper, she will have the staff connect her to her children by phone. Her discipline poses a problem to caregivers who are not used to that style. Before we join the trend of many who believe that she has OCPD, let's remember what Alfred Adler taught us. Before we judge a man or a woman, we should know what environment they grew up in. Mrs. Red was born in Germany and grew up in a culture that celebrates discipline as a tradition. Mrs. Red simply is not used to and cannot function in chaos. It became clear from the chaplain's point of view that the staff needed to hear this information. Concerned about Mrs. Red's mental health due to constant frustration, he felt it was imperative to reconcile Mrs. Red and the staff as a spiritual intervention.

Mrs. Brown has been in hospice for the last eight months. She is dependent on diagnosing senile degeneration of the brain. Confused but relatively silent most of the time, however, at 3:00 pm every day, Mrs. Brown becomes restless, anxious, and shouts at the staff that she needs to take the bus to get to work. When asked why she wants to take the bus, she always responds that her boss will punish her if she is not on time. She exhibits genuine fear talking about her boss. Probably, Mrs. Brown had a difficult boss or supervisor while she was active professionally. Her trauma (PTSD) is obvious.

However, should we turn to Freud to explain that behavior or to Carl Gustav Jung? From a Freudian perspective, this is the re-surgence of what was unconscious. But the question becomes: is Mrs. Brown's fear a repressed element? With that, Mrs. Brown's advanced dementia stage, the "shadow" of Carl Gustav Jung helps explain her condition. The "mask" is off, and the archetype developed during the professional years is resurfacing as the content of Mrs. Brown's shadow. She is now 85, and her fear of her boss is still alive and well, and the habit of taking the bus at 3:00 pm hasn't left her. In her moments of lucidity, Mrs. Brown likes many in the facility.

Depression is common with almost all the residents. However, Uncle Dean is also a man with a sense of humor. Former Elite in the Army, he takes pride in recounting his years in service. He lost his wife two years ago, and he is still grieving. After 70 years of marriage, Uncle Dean felt that he had lost one part of himself. Yet, he still comes to the breakfast early in the morning with some of the residents. Uncle Dean fits John H. Morgan's description in the theory of geriatric narcissism and the late-life geriatric depression between reminiscence and grief.

Often at the early breakfast table, Father Blue, a former French literature professor from a local university appears, but not because he's famished. He's an intellectual addicted to knowledge and intellectual debate. He is always happy when he has the opportunity to speak French and engage in an intellectual debate. At 96, he is cognizant and independent. As if he read Dr. Morgan about geriatric narcissism, he complains about the usual discussion among the residents. He confides that they only talk about their achievements, how great they were, and how deprived is the current generation. Every discussion is the indictment of the new generation. He once said in French: "Je ne Suis pas fou." Fr. Blue knows that many around him have a sort of dementia, advanced or mild, and/or memory loss. At 96, he is older than many and still totally independent. However, he has some 'older sisters' around.

Mrs. Kay is 101 years old, also totally independent and very assertive. One day, their lunch location was moved to the basement. She objected, saying, though she can walk independently, many could not have moved that easily, for they were in a wheelchair. While the administrator who made the decision was standing there, she asked loudly: "Who made that stupid decision?" There was total silence. Mrs. Kay has reached that age when one can say almost anything without real objection from the staff. Geriatric narcissism or not, after 100 years of age, she has earned that right.

Mrs. Avon, also, at 102, is not impressed with anything. When she smiles, that is the exception. But unlike Mrs. Kay, she is dependent, which explains her frustration and chronic depression. She and others seem to be annoyed by Mrs. Cup. Mrs. Cup's baseline is to cry, as she becomes hysterical from time to time. She has dementia, but before that, she lost her husband and her two sons. It is when that memory resurfaces in her brain that she becomes hysterical. What is in the sub-conscious is resurfacing. She was born in Italy, and during her hysterical moments, she stops speaking in English and only speaks Italian. That complicated behavior brings us again to the dilemma about who explains best the attitude of Mrs. Cup. Though the subconscious seems to resurface, with the dementia diagnosis the "shadow" of Carl Jung helps us to understand that the "mask" of Mrs. Cup is off, and her shadow is revealing that grief and pain of hers. The attending physician prescribed some medication to control that behavior totally; however, the chaplain cautioned against taking that moment away. The chaplain explained that it is a moment of remembrance. "Instead of putting her on medication, why don't we let her vent that emotion for the two to three minutes it usually lasts? She is already in hospice, and it is her new normal."

Like Mrs. Cup, Mrs. Pen, her roommate, is also in hospice. Mrs. Pen is nonverbal. Musical tune and piano keyboard become the way of communication between the chaplain and Mrs. Pen. After learning about her favorite playlist, chaplain resumed using that as a communication tool. After few weeks in, Mrs. Pen, though nonverbal, shows motions and vibration while listening to songs. Her eyes sometimes become brighter, after what the chaplain calls liturgical pastoral care.

On the other side near the nursing station, Mrs. Iron stands near the nursing station's counter. Mrs. Iron used to be a supervisor in a local hospital kitchen. Though she has advanced dementia, she always stood at the nursing station with a serious demeanor as a supervisor controlling workflow.

Mrs. Eve was a friend with many residents. Five of them passed one after another. At the age of 87, she confided to the chaplain that she is aware of that reality (death), but "I am not prepared for it," she said. In the same recreational room, Mr. Rough is relatively young, in his early 60s. He has multiple co-morbidity and is in a wheelchair. He is losing parts of his body, as they are being amputated due to infections. Mr. Rough has developed a deep sense of theodicy. In his case, Viktor Frankl and his will to meaning have proven effective in that palliative approach of containing his emotions and walking through this process, one day, one step at a time. Frankl became important to

Mr. Rough as it speaks to human nature's resiliency in the face of affliction.

Mrs. Eve was removed and admitted to the hospital a few days ago. Her absence in the activity room is noticeable. Many residents are used to that routine. Someone suddenly disappears. But officially, the news of Mrs. Eve's death was broken to the group. And there was silence, silence that translates the thoughts of many residents of long-term care facilities.

Everyone is wondering, who will be next? Each person is conscious of death's reality and knows that they are walking through that valley of the shadow of death.

As we talk about Carl Jung and Freud and their understanding of certain behaviors, let's briefly mention their thoughts in that regard.

Talking about patient's resistance, Freud wrote that:

"We told the patient that he should without further reflection put himself into a condition of calm and self-observation. They must then communicate whatever results this introspection gives him—feelings, thoughts, reminiscences, in which they appear to his mind." He then continued, "At the same time, we warn him expressly against yielding to any motive which would induce him to choose or exclude any of his thoughts as they arise. In whatever way, the motive may be couched, and however, it may excuse him from telling us his thoughts: 'that is too pleasant' it is 'nonsensical.' We impress upon him that he must skim only across the surface of his consciousness and toward that which he finds. We finally inform him that the result of the treatment and, above all, its length is dependent on the conscientiousness with which he follows this basic rule of the analytic technique. According to Freud, the patient directs her entire resistance against it. The patient tries in every way to escape it. Compulsive neurotics are exceedingly adept at making this technical rule almost useless by bringing to bear all their over-consciousness and their doubts upon it. Patients suffering from anxiety-hysteria sometimes succeed in reducing it to absurdity by producing only notions so remote from the things sought for that analysis is quite unprofitable."

While in the collective unconsciousness, Carl Gustav Jung wrote that:

The persona: it is a mask that individuals put on in response to demands required of the social environment and tradition and consort with their own archetypal needs. This is the role the community constructs and expects them to play. Mental illness appears when conflict arises.

The anima and the animus: are generally recognized in all psychological science branches as indicative of the bisexual nature. Physiologically, the human-animal secretes both male and female sex hormones, and on the psychological level, masculine and feminine characteristics are found in both sexes.

For Jung, "Man apprehends the nature of woman

by her animus. Mental illness results when there is an imbalance.

The 'shadow' is "the most ancient of the archetypes and originates from the lowest forms of evolutionary life which we have inherited, and therefore, the shadow typifies the animal nature of man more than any other and expresses itself in images and ideas of evil, the devil's wickedness, and the enemy. These constitute feeling-based content..." It is the dark side of the controlled ego and personality that must have the energy which is derived from the shadow just as it must have the energy derived from the images of the other archetypes such as mother and wise old man.

The 'self' is "the center of personality, and all other human mind components form a circling constellation around it. It holds the mental structure in place, providing unity, equilibrium, and stability to the individual's state of mind. The self functions as an archetype and constitutes the goal of every person striving for a sense of self.

Freud speaks to the neurotic patient with certain capacities which are fully capable, though with memory loss and dementia. The unconscious reveals itself, but with less resistance, as the persons are not fully in control of their loss of the "Self." Jung is not in contrast with Freud; his belief seems to complete the Freudian theory by providing the patients' state of mind. Jung allows us to explain that the mask is off, and the human shadow drives the behavior.

Unquestionably, the changes people experience

in their late-life lead to various personality changes, mental health issues, and in extreme cases, personality disorder. It is what geriatric psychotherapy is trying to explain and palliate.

II

A case for spiritual care (With Carl Gustav Jung)

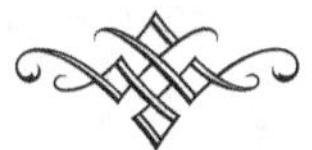

Psychotherapy or Clergy

Carl Jung once wrote that "it is the urgent psychic problem of patients, much more than the questions posed by scientific workers which has given effective impetus to the newer developments in medical psychology and psychotherapy. Jung stated that "the science of medicine has avoided all contact with strictly psychic problems. It has held to this position despite the patients' urgent needs. For Jung, it was natural that a "new direction should be given to these adopted branches of science." He further gave an example of psychiatry. It helped, he says, itself out of the treasure chest of experimental psychology. He also stated that "it funded its borrowing in that inclusive body of knowledge called psychopathology." Jung believes that "psychology is built for one part upon the findings of psychiatry in the straight sense of the term and the other upon the findings of neurology a field of study which originally embraced the so-called psychogenetic neuroses, and still does so in academic parlance. However, in practice, Jung wrote, a gulf has opened in the last few years between the trained neurologist and the psychotherapist. This rift, he continues, "is traceable to the first researches in hypnotism." He suggested, "Investigation established beyond the crux of psycho-neuroses is to find the psychic factor. This is the essential cause of the pathological state and must therefore be recognized in its own right along with other admitted pathogenic factors such as inheritance, disposition, bacterial infection and so forth." Jung realized that all attempts to explain the psychic factor in terms of more elementary physical factors were doomed to failure." The question Jung asks is: What could seem more plausible, therefore, than to seek the specific cause of the psycho-neuroses, not in the mystical notion of the soul, but in a disturbance of the impulses which might be curable in the last resort by medicinal treatment of the glands?

He then pointed out Freud's standpoint when establishing his well-known theory which explains neuroses in terms of disturbances of the urge to power. Adler likewise, he continued, resorts to the concept of the drive and explains neuroses in terms of disturbances of the urge to power." On this basis, he thinks that "psychic factor is just a combination of instincts which for their part may again be reduced to the functioning of the glands. "We may," he continues, "even discuss the possibility that everything that is usually called psychic is embraced in the sum-total of instinct or a conglomerate of instinct." In contrast, he affirms that "on the other hand, we have been taught by all too many mistakes that organic medicine fails in the treatment of neuroses, while psychic methods cure them." He then made it clear that "It is no reproach to the Freudian and Adlerian theories that they are based upon the drives; the only trouble is that they are one-sided. The kind of psychology they represent leaves out the psyche and is suited to people who believe that they have no spiritual needs or aspirations. In this matter, both doctors and patients deceive themselves. He explains that "it fails because of their exclusive concern with the drives to satisfy the patients' deeper spiritual needs." He advises physicians to refer clients to a clergyman and the philosopher." According to Jung, human thought cannot conceive any system or final truth that could give the patient what he needs to live: that is faith, hope, love, and insight." These are the four highest achievements of human effort and many gifts of grace, which are neither taught nor learned, neither given nor taken, neither withheld nor earned; they come through experience, which is something given beyond the reach of human caprice. Experience, Jung wrote, cannot be manufactured; experiences simply happen. Jung then wondered how he could help a sufferer attain the liberating experience that will bestow upon him four great gifts of grace and heal his sickness. He noted then that "Protestant clergymen often find themselves face to face with an almost impossible task, for they have to cope with practical difficulties that the Catholic priest is spared. Talking about psychology without psychic, Jung stated that the reason given for not consulting the church minister was generally his lack of psychological knowledge and insight. "What is the meaning of my life or life in general? he asked. Jung reflected by saying, "I have found that modern man has an ineradicable aversion to traditional opinions and inherited truths. He is the Bolshevist whose spiritual standards and forms have lost their validity and want to experiment in the world of spirits as the Bolshevist experiments with economics. He continues, "Some people no longer feel themselves to have been redeemed by the death of Christ. They cannot seem to believe, and they cannot compel themselves to believe, however happy they may deem the human who has a belief. Sin has, for them, become something quite relative. Can what is evil for one be good for the other?"

After all, why should not Buddha be in the right also? For Jung, disturbance in the sphere of the unconscious drives is not primary but secondary phenomena. When conscious life has lost its meaning and promise, it is as though panic has broken loose, and we hear the exclamation, 'Let us eat and drink, for tomorrow we die!' Jung suggested that "it is this mood, born of the meaninglessness of life that causes the disturbance in the unconscious and provokes the painfully curbed impulses to break out anew. Therefore the cause of neurosis lies in the present as well as in the past." By consequence, "This is why I regard the religious problems which the patient brings before me as relevant to the neurosis and as possible causes of it." Speaking against condemnation, he said that it does not liberate; it oppresses. Jung defines neurosis as a dissociation of the personality. To the psychotherapist, Jung suggested they must come to grips with these questions. They must decide in every simple case whether or not they are willing to stand by a human being with counsel and help upon what may be an actual misadventure. He must have no fixed ideas as to what is right and what is not. Otherwise, he takes something from the richness of the experience. If something that seems to be an error shows itself to be more effective than truth, then I must first follow up the error, for it lies power and life, which I lose if I hold to what seems to be true. "Light has need of darkness—otherwise how could it appear as light? "Freud," Jung wrote, "overlooked that man has never yet been able single-handedly to hold his own against the power of darkness that is unconscious." Jung concluded this chapter by stating, "Medicine man is also the priest, he is the savior of the body as well as the soul and religions are systems of healing for psychic illness."

The apple didn't fall far from the tree. Jung, a son of a pastor and grandson of a pastor, followed Kant's footstep to not alienate their faith in the midst of intellectual reflection. This chapter, however, addresses some of the questions I faced in pastoral care practice. How can we neglect the spiritual dimension of people? In the wake of the 2008 crisis and the new health care laws implementation, it was an open season on pastoral care. The first department dismantled in most hospitals was pastoral care. Clinical Pastoral Education was suppressed, and the number of chaplains reduced. It happened that in my journey as a chaplain, I worked with people in the early stages of disabilities—people with various faiths and belief systems; Judaism, Christianity, Islam, Buddhism, and atheism. The observation is that the people who believe have a better coping system than those who do not. For example, Christians who believe that a God Almighty, strong enough to take them out of their situations, felt a huge weight lifted off their shoulders. It was the same thing with Judaism and Islam.

In contrast, it wasn't easy with Buddhism and atheism because the philosophy of the belief is based on self-achievement. The Buddhists and the atheists faced a challenge in that circumstance; their bodies are incapacitated and unable to function and are in stocks. In this case, the belief placed in a Mighty God is helpful; it helps alleviate the weight and the anxiety of these patients. Spirituality in patients' lives is overlooked because most people think that the chaplain's job is limited to the recitation of "The Lord's Prayer."

In the end of life situation, where patients are

in comfort measure only, I have tried to explain to nurses, physicians, and social workers that everybody has their own spirituality. I think that everybody has their own spirituality like we all have our own personality. Even in the same congregation, some people are lifted spiritually by worship, hymnal, sermon, or the fellowship. Spirituality can be diagnosed and pinpointed like any other human dimension. At the end of life, or hospice, there is rarely psychiatric involvement in the care. Chaplains often fill that role. Doing so, we should assess with precision what is the source of spiritual comfort of giving individuals. That spiritual comfort is everything that uplifts the spirit of individuals and provides them with peace of mind and well-being in the soul. This spirituality can be found at church or near a glass of Johnny Walker. The individual who finds happiness in watching the Giants game on Sunday morning seeks to cultivate spirituality like the person who finds solace in Sunday morning worship. The difference is that the trust in God, who made heaven and earth fulfills their spirits, while the spectacle on the field helps other individual spirits. Jung, critic of the Protestant clergyman, is real. In the church, the assumption of homogeneity of spirituality can be overlooked. However, at the end of life, hospice, defining the precise spirituality is essential as the mental strength is decreasing. It is quintessential to pinpoint the individuals' spirituality to their favorite hymn, favorite scripture, and in the case of many people who embrace faith as a culture (cultural Jews and Christian) to identify what nourishes their spirits. Even though I agree with Jung that Catholic priests have fewer problems than the Protestant clergyman, there are some limitations. There are unquestionably certain psychological benefits of the Sacrament of The Sick for people. Catholic chaplain presence and touch are enough for most patients. When a priest enters a hospital room, it is a sense of relief for the Catholic patient. In the case of end of life, the Sacrament of the Sick provides the individual with a certain assurance to make it to "Our Father's House." However, observation shows that the fear of the unknown persists. The Sacrament of the Sick indeed provides relief to the family of the patient, but most patients carry with them the fear of the unknown. At that precise moment, it becomes helpful to explore and identify the spirituality of the individuals. What gives them genuine hope? What nourishes their spirits?

For this reason, extensive psychological training should be added to the curriculum at the seminary. A clergy without psychology and Clinical Pastoral Education has incomplete training. Alcoholics Anonymous is an example of psychology integrated into theology.

Adler and Freud's theories are incomplete to the critic because of a lack of theological integration or failure to address individuals' spiritual dimension. It is important to put this in context. In Adler, Freud, Karl Marx, the leaderships of the major religions were viewed as oppressors. For this reason many stayed away and were careful to address people's spirituality. Karl Marx even calls it the 'people's opioid.' Voltaire earlier stayed away from religion to freely express his viewpoint. Jung's criticism of Adler and Freud shows the theological differences between cultural Jews and a practicing Protestant Swiss. Though Freud and Adler were not fans of religion, the message of Grace and Redemption in the Christian faith carries a psychological dimension beyond our understanding. The guilt that is taken away by the redemptive story is important. The question will then be, are Adlerian and Freudian theories helpful to a patient filled with guilt. While the absolution given by the priest is valuable, as well as the sermon on grace preached by a Protestant preacher, it is still unclear how well the Adlerian and the Freudian methods can help in that circumstance.

III

Review of Geriatric psychology literature

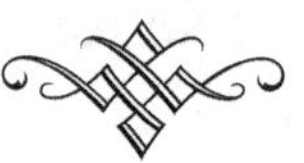

(THE EXTENSIVE WORK OF DR. JOHN H. MORGAN
AND OTHERS ON GERIATRIC PSYCHOLOGY)

Retirement & Mental Health

This chapter encompasses a decade of research and review presented by Dr. John H. Morgan in his book "Geriatric Psychotherapy, "the eleventh chapter.

John H. Morgan wrote that 'Over thirty years ago, Rosen and Palmer (1982) raised the issue of the relationship between professional women's notion of themselves and their attitude toward retirement.

That lecture essay was significant, at least in terms of its early call for a more sophisticated study of this phenomenon, which, alas, has yet to be thoroughly studied using evidence-based data.

Rosen and Palmer, in that regard, contended that the psychosocial consequences of this transition had at the time received very little attention, and we might suggest that even today, this is a very much under-studied correlation.

However, they discovered that most interviewees were satisfied with their lives, but they report that a substantial minority suggested periodic restlessness or boredom.

Those who reported being dissatisfied with retirement indicated negative and ambivalent feelings and anxiety regarding filling the void in their lives upon retirement.

Rosen and Palmer's hypothesis was that women's self-concept over a lifetime constitutes the best single predictor of successful retirement adjustment.

Pitt (1990) pointed to the conspicuous absence of evidence-based studies linking retirement to mental illness. He did, however, point out that retirement may contribute a little to depression, neurosis, subjective anxiety, and marital tension."

Pitt concluded by suggesting a range of attitudes and activities that may promote successful retirement, including physical activities and mental activities.

Fletcher and Hanson (1991) used the Retirement Anxiety Scale (SCRAS), social components in a series of four studies involving 308 men and 384 women aged 25 to 76 years testing for retirement anxiety.

The result of the scale assessment of responses demonstrated a strong prediction of fear of retirement and a negative attitude toward it.

However, it failed in its ability to measure a generalized emotional state, demonstrated simply a rather minimal correlation with other more generalized measurements of anxiety and depression.

Nearly 20 years ago, Sharpley (1997) did the psychological research community a favor by addressing psychometric properties related to self-perceived stress on what was then called the Retirement Scale.

That study showed a structured configuration demonstrating three factors of relevance in anxiety and depression induction, including missing work, personal health, and relationship issues.

Kim and Moen (2002) pursued a longitudinal study of the relationship between retirement and post-retirement psychological well-being, a topic of great interest.

Their study strongly suggests that understanding the dynamics of retirement transition related to psychological well-being must inevitably be linked to a study of the context within the retirement transition. They believed that gender, prior level of psychological well-being, spouses' circumstances, and changes in personal control marital quality, subjective health, and income adequacy must be considered fundamental factors.

Melzer (2004) and colleagues addressed the widespread issue of the common mental disorder prevalence among older men in their 60s based on their assessment of the data gleaned in the National Psychiatric

Morbidity Survey.

Melzer and team concluded that: within the general population aged 50-74 years, there is a measurable boost in mental health among men after the traditional retirement age of 65 but not among women. However, for men who leave work earlier than the traditional age of 65, the prevalence of mental disorders remains somewhat high until the age of 65, when depressive symptoms recede.

Togas (2004) and colleagues have taken on a commonly held negative view of older workers and their relationship to identity and relative deprivation related to ageism and retirement.

They confirmed their hypothesis by showing that the end-of-career experiences directly impact the retirees' post-retirement life situation.

They suggest that the more these young retirees integrate aging workers' characteristics, the more they feel deprived of their younger co-workers. Self-esteem and the assessment of one's life satisfaction declined markedly as well.

Karankawa (2005) and colleagues addressed themselves about depression brought on by early retirement.

The study results were clear; a high depression score predicted disability due to any cause, especially mental disorders and non-illness-based pensions. Depressed individuals retired on average a year and a half younger than those without depression. Further study is justified in charting the pathways of how mental depression leads workers to seek retirement pension.

Butterworth (2006) and colleagues in a substantial national research project on retirement in Australia indicated the sparsity of such evidence-based empirical investigations is a major concern in the national health community.

This study's findings indicated that the relationship between retirement and mental health increase with age but less so with women. Butterworth and team believe that these findings should encourage weighing mental health issues and their influencing factors when encouraging continued employment among older adults, especially men.

Villani, Huppert, and Melzer (2006) have produced a remarkable data-based study linking depression and anxiety to retirement based on a national survey conducted in the United Kingdom.

"Anxiety disorders registered a lower prevalence for men at 80% and women at 50%, and not surprisingly, men's work status proved significant but not for women.

Srinivas and Davey (2006) broke new ground on a topic that was beginning to dominate social service agencies, namely the relationship between depression and grandchild care among retirees. Srinivas and Davey's conclusion based on this study suggests that the traditional argument that family care obligations spoil the retirement year proved correct for men. For women, the case was not made for such a conclusion but rather to the contrary.

Karelia (2011) and colleagues set out to study a virtually unstudied classification of workers, namely employees who have personality disorders and the relevance of that classification to retirement issues compared to anxiety and depression.

They concluded that: personality disorders increase the risk of early retirement at about the same level as depression but more than twice that of anxiety disorders.

Bekhet and Azuszniewski (2013) addressed themselves to the issue of cross-cultural differences concerning the aging process and the adjustments to it with a specific interest in a comparative study of the United States and Egypt since both older populations are expected to double by the year 2030.

The study's benefit offered a direction for developing positive cognition intervention methods and engaging older individuals in the decision-making process to adjust to relocation.

The study's specific relevance offered suggestions on how residential facilities' nursing staff might assist in the positive thinking and resourcefulness training required. These interventions have proven beneficial in reducing relocation stress by facilitating positive thinking about the inevitability of relocation.

Potocnik and Sonnentag (2013) find that "there is a rise in depression among both retirees and older employees who were directly involved in the care of disabled adults.

For instance, cases in which retirees were suffering

from higher levels of depression, participation in religious activities resulted in a greater decrease in depression than those who were suffering at a lower level of depression. An additional finding was that older employees who took an active part in political activities experienced a decrease in depression.

Chli, Stewart, and Dewey (2013) did a large data-based study of the relationship between variously identified productive activities and the prevalence of depression among a large sampling of older Europeans.

Chli and the team concluded that formalized volunteering activities might be somewhat important in reducing depression and the risk of developing depressive symptoms. Nevertheless, caregiving is rather directly associated with a higher risk of depression with older European adults.

Paunio (2014) and colleagues concluded from their study that poor sleeping patterns are important data in the etiology of both depression and resulting disability retirement. They concluded this information should encourage both early detection and treatment of sleep disturbances and poor quality sleep patterns.

"Stan Cliffe (2014) and colleagues found that: "the use of trained mentors in community social groups is a viable option for developing a retirement lifestyle for individuals anticipating disabilities.

Airagnes (2014) and colleagues affirmed that studies in advance have consistently shown that a positive effect of retirement is manifested in depressive symptoms.

Airagnes and colleagues concluded that individuals with a high level of cognitive hostility were more likely to demonstrate less improvement in depressive symptoms following retirement versus those in the lowest level of cognitive hostility.

Ladin, Daniels, and Kawachi (2014) concluded that mental health disparities throughout later life where individuals are exposed to higher levels of national inequality experience greater morbidity than those in countries with less inequality.

Ghodsbin and colleagues concluded that laughter therapy has proven to have practical benefits in general health among the elderly despite its lack of positive impact upon depression.

Lohman (2015) and colleagues showed a very high level of significant correlation between depression and the various models of frailty factors and depressive biological syndrome, functional domains, and frailty index.

Psychological vulnerability may very well be a key factor in frailty among the elderly.

A study by Grotz (2015) and colleagues suggest a measurable relationship between retirement age and the age of the onset of Alzheimer's disease. There is extreme caution in overvaluing these findings due to the selection bias of participants and uncertainty in the causality correlation, leading the researchers to suggest that further study is mandatory to more positively clarify and validate the relevance of these findings.

Olsen (2015) and colleagues have further explained

a very complex yet-to-be thoroughly studied relationship between retirement and mental health. Olsen (2015) and colleagues concluded that the massive data-based study did not and could not confirm their initial hypothesis that retirement is beneficial for mental health using as a measurement both hospitalizations caused by depression and treatment of depression with antidepressant medication.

Palliative Psycho-therapeutic: Option in Geriatric Depression Management

According to Dr. John H. Morgan, "neither psych-therapeutic nor biological psychiatry has made a name for itself in developing new approaches to the treatment of depression among the palliative care patient community."

However, according to Fairman, "what is now being called palliative care psychiatry is on the rise as an emerging sub-specialty where palliative methods converge (Fairman &Irwin, 2013)

Dr. Morgan wrote in that regard: "the interfacing of palliative care medicine with psychiatry is being heralded throughout the medical community as a positive step forward in the development of modalities of treatment. Both pharmacologically and psycho-therapeutically, which may be further researched and evidence-based tested for efficacy."

"Palliative psychotherapeutic care has, in recent years, become an increasingly important component of comprehensive health care treatment options.

There are, according to Karel and colleagues, "a large number of counselors and psychotherapists as well as psychiatrists, however, who find themselves with an increase in post-retirement clients and patients but without the benefit of specific training in treating this particular constituency (Karel, Ogland-Hand, Gatz, and Unuetzer, 2002, Gatz, Fiske, Fox, Kaskie, Kasl-Godley and McCallum, 1999, Hinrichsen, 2008)

Stanley and colleagues stated that: "there is a large population of older individuals in need of assistance in dealing with depression and its cognates of anxiety and self-esteem issues which are of particular concern to the health care professionals working in palliative care medicine (Stanley, Wilson, Nery, Rhodes, Wagener, Greisinger, 2009, Knight and MacCallum, 1998)

Gallagher and colleagues stated that "there is a relative void in the training of palliative care health professionals in geriatric psychotherapy, particularly as related to the treatment of depression. This is very evident according to recent AMA-sponsored studies (Gallagher-Thompson and Steffen, 1994).

This essay's interest is rather to call attention to several proven modalities of treatment available for non-medically trained psychotherapists dealing with palliative psychogenic depression (Knight & Qualls, 2006).

According to Francis and Kumar, "there are several modalities of treatment for late-life depression for both institutionalized patients and those living at home. (Francis & Kumar, 2013) This includes cognitive and behavioral therapy, problem-solving therapy, reminiscence and life review, brief psychodynamic therapy, and interpersonal therapy.

According to Herholz, consistent, evidence-based studies show that non-pharmacological interventions offer the prospect and the improvement of psychosocial aspects of older individuals suffering from mild cognitive impairment Alzheimer's dementia. (Herholz, Herholz, Herholz, 2013)

"Recent studies will be reviewed here including those involving cognitive training and reminiscence and also such components as visual art and music, physical activities, and electro-magnetic stimulation."

Specific treatment modalities which evidence-based effectiveness record to date include Cognitive Behavior Therapy (Barrowclough, King, Colville, Russell, Burns, and Tarrier, 2001, Cappeliez, 2001; Siskin, 2002)

"Brief Dynamic Therapy (Messer, 2001)

"Interpersonal Psychotherapy (Hinrichsen & Clougherty, 2006)

"Reminiscence Therapy (Bohlmeijer, Smit, and Cuijpers, 2003)

"Geriatric Logotherapy (Morgan, 2012)

"Behavioral Therapies, particularly Cognitive Behavioral Therapy (CBT) and Rational

Emotive Behavior Therapy (REBT), have been the most used modalities of treating non-medical or psychogenic depression among older clients and have the largest data-based evidence for effectiveness (Floyd & Scogin, 1998).

"Depression is considered within the cognitive-behavioral school of psychotherapy to essentially constitute the inability of the individual to cope with stress brought on by the aging process itself."

"That includes problem-solving skills isolation within the social matrix of daily living and the decline in physical skills capabilities."

"The emphasis in these CBT treatment options focuses upon the practicalities of skill enhancement and the intentionality in the reorientation toward life stressors by reconfiguring the client's daily schedule, priorities, and inclination (Gatz, 2007).

"The CBT agenda is two-fold, to reduce the psychogenic depression and elevate the social interaction and the physical skills-based functioning of the client. Reducing depressive behavior while increasing social and physical activity constitutes the treatment agenda of CBT, and evidence for its effectiveness is substantial." CBT has a longevity value beyond that of pharmacological treatments (Hyer,

Hilton, Sacks, Freidman, and Yeager).

The various factors of methodological limitations, protective attitudes of healthcare providers, and the progressive deterioration of patients with terminal disease have heretofore proven effective deterrents to evidence-based studies.

One area in which palliative care medical practice has only just begun to address itself is the realization that since half of the cancer patients today continue to die of the disease, there is inevitably a persistence of psychological distress associated with it.

According to Japan Oncology Society (Akechi, 2010), Oncology patients frequently develop adjustment disorders and debilitating depression, including anticipatory nausea and vomiting for patients receiving melogenic chemotherapeutic agents.

The amelioration of depression within the palliative care treatment patient using evidence-based effective psychotherapies constitutes the health caregiver's agenda and the institutional support team of medical personnel.

Studies (Connell, 1998) are now regularly providing evidence-based data to validate Reminiscence Therapy's effectiveness (RT) used to treat geriatric depression within the nursing home institutional setting. RT is a non-pharmacological intervention involving the prompting of memories on memories of palliative care patients.

The most prevalent mental health disorder among

institutionalized elderly is depression. Studies demonstrate the common usage of RT in the treatment of dementia care showing effective results in the enhancement of self-esteem and improved communication skills, self-worth, personal identity, and sense of individuality.

Reminiscence Therapy (RT) benefits for improving the quality of life of individuals, both in and out of institutionalized care facilities, suffering from dementia, have consistently produced evidence-based validation.

Despite the frequency of reports regarding effectiveness in the use of Reminiscence Therapy (RT) in the treatment of depression and dementia among the institutionalized elderly population (Klever, 2013), there is a conspicuous absence of actual evidence addressing the specifics of the connection between reminiscence functions and the reduction of depressive symptoms (Hallford, Mellor, & Cummings, 2013).

As a variation of Reminiscence Therapy, Group Reminiscence Therapy is commonly used within a group of aged peers suffering from psychogenic depression in an institutional setting such as a residential nursing home.

Problem-Solving Therapy (PST) (Kiosses & Alexopoulos, 2004) is a component of geriatric psychogenic depression treatment. It is consistently reporting an evidence-based effectiveness rate justifying both its continued use and further data-collection and assessment.

"Used with patients suffering from minor depression as well as dysthymia (especially stroke patients)

Meaning-Centered Group Psychotherapy (MCGP) is increasingly becoming recognized as a legitimate treatment modality addressing the spiritual and values-based world-view of the terminally ill and end-of-life elderly palliative care patient (Breithart, Rosenfeld, Gibson, Pessin, Poppito, Nelson, Tomarken, Timm, Berg, Jacobson, Sorger, Abbey, and Olden, 2010).

Mindfulness-Based Supportive Therapy (MBST) is addressed particularly to palliative psychotherapy employed in the treatment of psycho-existential suffering of the end-of-life patient."

The MBST consists of five key components, viz. presence, listening, empathy, compassion, and boundary awareness (Beng, Chin, Guan, Yee, Wu, Jane and Meng, 2013)

Dignity Therapy (DT)

It is a brief psychotherapeutic modality treatment for depression and anxiety for the institutionalized elderly with a terminal illness, where palliative caregivers evidence a high level of distress.

Existential Behavioral Therapy (EBT) was developed to support palliative patients' informal caregivers in the last stage of life. During bereavement, manualized group therapy consists of six sessions only (Febb, Brandstatter, Kogler, Hauke, Rechenberg-winter, Fensterer, Kuchenhoff, Hentrich, Belka, and Borasio, 2013).

Forgiveness Therapy is now beginning to provide evidence-based validation of its efficacy in improving psychological well-being on the part of the patient and promises to be a valuable component of terminal care treatment plans (Hansen, Enright, Baskin and Klatt, 2009).

They measure such things as forgiveness, hope, quality of life, and anger issues.

Palliative psychotherapy is a fairly recent arrival in the care and treatment of the terminally ill and particularly geriatric institutionalized patients suffering from debilitating depression.

Suggestion of Geriatric Logo therapy as Depression treatment option
- The notion of Geriatric Logotherapy

Logotherapy is a type of psychotherapeutic analysis and treatment that focuses on a 'will to meaning.' It is founded upon the belief that striving to find meaning in one's life is the primary, most powerful motivation and driving force within the human experience sometimes called existential analysis (Frank, 1967, 2002).

-Pastoral Logotherapy applies logotherapeutic analysis and treatment within the context of Spiritual understanding of the human situation and its relevance to mental health.

Geriatric Logotherapy is then a sub-set of this analytical approach designed to address issues uniquely confronted in the pastoral encounter with the elderly.

According to Frankl, life has meaning under all circumstances, even in the direst situation. "What matters is not the meaning of life in general," Frankl suggested, "but rather the specific meaning of a person's life at a given moment. Meaning is not 'invented' but rather 'detected'."

He points out that "we can discover meaning in life in three different ways: (1) By doing a deed; (2) by experiencing a value-nature, a work of art, another person's love, etc., and by suffering.

For Frankl, three fundamental human existence characteristics converge to define the human person, namely spirituality, freedom, and responsibility.

This tripartite foundation inevitably affects every attempt to understand who we are and what we are to do.

Frankl believes that any model of psychotherapeutic analysis and treatment must have a strong philosophical basis (Frankl, 1961b). "Where religious world view and ethos stifle, cripple, or delude an individual, Frankl is opposed to it."

A deeply felt sense of beauty, power, and wonder in the universe, a heightened experience of integrality, what Dr. Morgan called 'systemic integrality?' constitute what spirituality means in Logotherapy (Morgan 2009).

This sense of spirituality in Logotherapy is the freedom that functions in the face of three things: (1) the instincts, (2) inherited disposition, and (3) the environment. To rise above one's instincts is a distinctively human possibility.

Frankl was not a member of the 'nurture" crowd of behavioral psychologists, who would attribute, or even blame one's social and physical environment for the way individuals turned out in their maturity. Besides spirituality and freedom, there is responsibility.

The three schools of thought regarding the origin of ethics and moral behavior are: naturally good, behavioral history of moral development (2005), and more specifically, the three schools as Ethical Theism, Ethical Humanism and Ethical Naturalism (beyond divine intervention)

When Logo-therapy is applied to the geriatric patient, there is a challenge to transform the therapeutic practice's central concepts to people's life situations whose lives have, for all practical purposes, lost hope.

The interpretive hermeneutic of pastoral Logotherapy, rather than focusing upon hope for a cure of the depression and ennui being experienced by the late-life patient, it focuses rather upon memories of times past, which bring a moment of reflective happiness now.

The intent is to explicate from an existential memory of happy recollection a deeper sense of the meaningfulness of life as lived in the moment.

This means that, in this therapeutic instance, it constitutes a matrix of converging memory and existential happiness. It provides a practical formula for therapeutic application when dealing with terminal patients so diagnosed and late-life depression patients whose cognitive functions offer a broader range of access to recollected memories.

The existential character of the remembered happy events constitutes the possibility for a treasure trove of episodic happy vignettes bringing comfort to the elderly facing a limited future.

Unlike other schools of thought, which too frequently presume to be the panacea for all mental disorders, Logotherapy has self-consciously identified its arenas of success and knows those in which it has little or no value.

When applied to the treatment of the elderly, not as curative but as palliative therapy, there is a promise of success.

IV

The End of Life Therapy

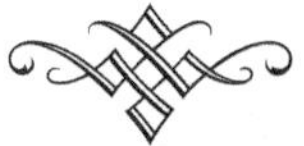

Grief and anticipatory grief in geriatric psychotherapy

The moment the seniors enter the nursing home or the long-term care facility to the moment of their death is a missing piece in our study. That stage in the life of the elderly is neither "geriatric ennui" nor something compared to a stage of death. It is a period when they lose their home or living quarters, the driver's license, the independence, sometimes their life partner. With almost no time for adjustment, they witness the passing of their new friends one after another in the facility. This is literally "walking through the valley of the shadow of death." The seniors are faced with the reality of their own mortality.

As they watch their peers passing, they wonder who is next. This may seem almost like being on "death row" and waiting for your turn. Viktor Frankl certainly knew the sentiments of being on death row waiting for your turn. The existential question about one's own destination becomes the cause of anticipatory grief, the root of depression. 'Where am I going from here?' is usually the question; however, the second is: where are they going? Affected by the fear of the unknown, the grief the elderly experience in that phase of life is somehow complicated. Most studies focus on retirement depression, but only a few on that stage of "walking through the valley of shadow of death. This moment or stage of life needs more academic studies. Addressing the senior's grief becomes important, for it is the root cause of their depression at that stage.

In that regard, as we anticipate the next book by Dr. Morgan, we can use a quote in this latest that is relevant to the topic of root-cause." It seems that we concentrate too much upon symptoms and concern ourselves too little with their cause. "In the words of Packer Palmer, it says, "When we tell our story, we become human." The geriatric narcissism developed by Dr. John H. Morgan is addressing that part of the elderly story that needs to be told. Instead of a negative connotation, this is rather positive. Reviewing their lives with positive regard for their achievement helps the mental state of the elderly. We suggested that grief should become the new reality of the elderly, as we choose a Copernican turn in that regard. The main question is: what kind of psychotherapy is needed to address that stage when the elderly is "walking through the valley of shadow of death?"

Clinical Pastoral Psychotherapy in Practice
The End of Life Spiritual Care

The End of Life Spiritual Care and psychotherapy can be challenging because of the general "unknown" and fear of the "unknown."

According to an anonymous author, "Dying is not a medical experience, but a human experience."

Even though the obvious is refuted, modern psychiatry is limited in the case of a nonverbal patient in hospice. The patient on comfort medication only and unable to "communicate verbally" becomes a challenge for the psychiatrist, almost out of reach of the physician as the care is only for comfort. Nevertheless, the "human" entity is still present in that "body" and, in the absence of non-verbal communication, can still communicate through other human dimensions. In the face of this medical limitation, the question is how we care for these "non-verbal hospice patients. The extensive views of Dr. John H. Morgan in Clinical Pastoral Psychotherapy become important at this stage of life because they combine spirituality and psychotherapy. He wrote, "Clinical pastoral psychotherapy constitutes the practice of pastoral care conjoined with clinical therapy on the part of the ministry professional" (John H. Morgan 2012, p28).

At the end of life, with non-verbal patients, this

approach becomes necessary. I do agree that "there is no faith-based science, nor science-based faith." However, in that case, there is a vacuum that sciences have yet to cover.

Clinical pastoral psychotherapy might be the answer for that type of care; it considers all dimensions of a human being–the physical' and 'the spirits,' often abandoned by modern medicine.

The purpose of the End of Life Psychotherapy

Two major tools at the end of life are hospice care and or palliative care. The purpose of pastoral psychotherapy and/or pastoral care is to bring human experience to the dying process by caring for the emotional and the spiritual. This implies several types of care or processes: "Pastoral Nurturing of the Elderly, the 'Happy Memory; in Geriatric Logo-therapy (John H. Morgan, 2012, p 137), the use of the Ethics Committee as a venue for long-term Pastoral Care (John H. Morgan 2012, P121) "The Logic of the Spirits' as developed by James Lodder, finding the "Hidden Wholeness' (Palmer Parker).

With these considerations in mind, we can define 'end of life' spiritual care as the care that combines pastoral care and clinical psychotherapy to humanize the dying process. The end of life spiritual care comprises few methods of pastoral care and counseling. They are 'Ministry of Handshake,' the 'Wound Care therapy,' the 'End of Life Liturgies,' and the 'Liturgical

Pastoral Care.'

1. The Ministry of Handshake

Based on Dr. John H. Morgan's theory on nurturing the elderly through 'Happy Memory,' this is mostly intended for elders in long-term care facilities, especially in the dementia unit. Such ministry aims to reaffirm "the dignity of a human being" bringing happy memories to the elderly who often are subjected to medical routine for a while. The shaking hand ignites souvenirs of normal life and in doing so, speaks to human dignity.

The principle of the "Handshake" is based upon the fact that we do not often enter people's residence without a minimal civility, greeting, and acknowledgement. The long term care facility is the "residence" of these elderly, and they are to be acknowledged. This speaks to human dignity. I see this also as part of the concept of "happy memories" and nurturing elders in these memories. However, it is difficult to quantify the souvenirs that "Handshake" can bring to most people; however, the satisfaction of most patients and the honor of human dignity are clearly visible.

2. The "End of Life Liturgies."

The 'End of Life liturgies' ritual combines spiritual prayers, a song within the patient's belief system, and faith tradition. The 'End of Life liturgies' started as an alternative to the Sacrament of the Sick ritual in the absence of a Catholic priest, mostly Sunday at 11:00 am. There are fewer and fewer priests, and usually, the request for 'The Sacrament of the sick' Sunday morning between 10:00 am, and 11:00 am becomes a difficult request to fulfill. Facing that reality, the End of Life liturgy is offered to the actively dying patient and family. It is a combination of prayers and songs. The prayer is composed, taking into consideration the Jungian theory of removing the "mask" of oneself and to see the 'reality' of one's "shadow."

It speaks of hope yet does not deny the "pain' of the loss through Lamentations. The end of liturgy addresses the pain by recognizing the depths of human agony. It allows and gives individuals permission to grieve as it sets the tone for the grieving period. The finding in that regard is encouraging. Leading families through lamentations to face death's reality allows them to own the process as "theirs,' not as 'a strange circumstance.' The tears they shed become precious and meaningful and are considered fully as part of their new reality. Few lyrical songs are selected during the process.

3. The Liturgical Pastoral Care

Most non-verbal patients are usually discharged from pastoral care because of the inability to communicate, and if they are Catholic, the care is limited to last rites (Sacrament of the Sick)

After observing the non-verbal patient in the

memory care unit, I started what I now call "Liturgical Pastoral Care."

The principle is that the "human being" is present in that body in the absence of verbal communication. They can hear and communicate in different ways; instead of limiting communication to verbal interaction, I try to identify ways to communicate with every patient. The purpose of this action is to bring emotional and spiritual comfort to the patient.

After I get to know the non-verbal patient through observation and information from family and friends, religious views, favorite songs, favorite team, hymnal, and tunes, I proceed to the spiritual intervention called "bedside spiritual care."

For most religious people with ethos views of the world, it starts with a prayer within their tradition, a chant or hymns as I sit at their bedside. Then it continues with tunes and musical selections. Music expresses happiness more than sadness. After a few musical selections, I talk to the patient.

The result after that ritual differs from one patient to another. Some patients open their eyes, teary for a time, but wider; some try to move a part of their body. For some, you can feel a vibration within them in tune with the song, and for some the skin tone becomes brighter. In other words, there is a liveliness that the approach seems to generate in the patient.

From time to time, I proceed to play a plain musical instrument. A guitar player, I do not play piano at all. However, even just pressing the keyboard with a little harmony and staying away from total cacophony, patients respond by being attentive. Even when lethargic, they seem to gain some strength. This musical tool is not entertainment but rather a communication tool. These are the observations I have made till now. I do not have any definite conclusions at this time. However, I am encouraged by the result and what I observe, as it brings emotional and spiritual comfort to patients. I think about it as an application to the concept of "happy memories in geriatric Logotherapy."

4. The Wound Care Therapy

Wound care therapy is the emotional version of actual physical wound care. Grief and any brokenness is an emotional wound. Wound care consists of encouraging the patient to care for and bandage the emotional wound until the patient becomes comfortable with the loss and the grief is no longer disruptive in one's life.

The patient is given homework called "grieving time." This is time the patient sets aside weekly to grieve and go through the broken emotions. This homework is repeated till the patient becomes comfortable with the loss.

This wound care is based upon the Freudian suggestion of bringing the unconscious to the conscious. It also took some elements from Viktor Frankl as to how to turn the negative to the positive. By becoming comfortable with one's grief, we adhere to the spirit of Logotherapy by transforming the negative to the positive.

Wound care sessions comprise various activities that help the patient to bring the repressed emotions to the consciousness.

V

Our time of prayer and reflection

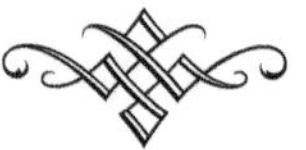

Our Time of Prayer and Reflection

It all started during a prayer service. It was a beautiful sunny day. We could see the blue sky from the window, with white clouds migrating from one place to another. The north's mild breeze was shaking the trees. Taking advantage of that beautiful day, wild turkeys took a walk through the little forest on the hill. There, a deer was running with a leaf in his mouth. Joining the show, the bluebirds were whistling to each other. What were they expressing? No one knows. But here in the room, the atmosphere was almost calm. The little tape near the chair of the chaplain was sending out the prelude. It was a lyric from Elvis, one of those oldies. It covered the room. The soft voice of Elvis was bringing the song directly into people's souls. The words were so familiar that we can hear the murmuring of the lyric, "You saw me cry in the chapel, the tears I shed were the tears of joy, now I know the meaning of contentment, and now I am happy with the Lord." While some were listening to the two lyrics, others were entering the room.

The calm of people brought serenity to the room. Everyone seemed to sing from the heart, calmly and peacefully. The expression of their eyes gave to their face the image of concerned and curious searchers. What were they thinking about? It was impossible to know. The music continued on the little tape to fulfill its mission by sending the message on its way.

Just at the end of the song, the chaplain broke the silence. "Good evening, everyone. Welcome to the time of prayer and reflection." All eyes were looking at him intently. He gave the outline of the meeting. He started the reading of the story of the day, The Ugly Duckling. As the story was read, the room looked like a third-grade classroom; sometimes, we could hear the people's breathing between pauses and periods. Then began the reflection: "Today," said the chaplain, "we heard about the ugly duckling who felt ugly because he differed from the others. Due to various circumstances when we find ourselves unable to move the way we used to when we find ourselves in a wheelchair, we think we look different from the rest of the world that we think is normal. We feel ugly like the little duckling. Are we ugly or does our comparison to others convince us that we are ugly? Our feeling is relative. When we compare ourselves to others, we might bring more pain to ourselves than is necessary.

The second thing in the story is the winter season. All was awkward during winter, but it saw a new day, a new chapter of its life when spring came. Sometimes we experience the same winter in our lives during which nothing seems to move for us. We experience a frozen time when the rhythm of our daily life slows down. As the chaplain was giving the reflection, a teary voice broke the silence.

"I don't want to be living in winter!" Patricia, one of the patients, was a middle-aged lady who seemed very strong despite her sitting in a wheelchair. We could see through her glasses a flow of tears falling. Patricia was at the end of the long table around which people were gathered. The other patients turned their faces toward her. The chaplain stopped, and the rest of the patients looked down toward the floor. The cries of Patricia took over the reflection. She continued, "I know that my life is frozen at this time, but I don't want to live like this. My winter is too long; I want my spring to come quickly."

All the people were astounded. The chaplain nodded his head to acknowledge what she was saying while the rest of the patients who happened to be older than the one who spoke put their hands near their faces and gave the impression of good listeners. All of a sudden, some of them started sharing in the tears.

And then she continued, "Chaplain, this winter is too long. I do not have the patience of Job. I want to get out of here and want to be at home. Do you think that God has something to do with this?" As she was sharing these words, almost all the patients were crying.

It was then that Cathy addressed her. Cathy was an elderly lady in her late nineties. She was always smiling, and passing through the alleys of the clinics, told some jokes and made everyone laugh. Though Cathy had a paralyzed hand, she seemed not to mind it. That day, Cathy seemed to have compassion for Patricia.

She looked up and began, "Patricia, I've had three strokes. I had breast cancer and now a hip replacement, but I am still here." After that introduction, everybody turned their attention to Cathy. All adjusted themselves to listen to her. From sad faces looking down, all turned their attention with more open faces, looking at her directly in the eyes. With all this attention, Cathy continued with a compassionate voice, "No one wants to be here, but what do you want to do now?"

At that question, Patricia replied: "I am not fine with my life. I'm tired of this life. I do not have the patience to endure all these things."

That answer made Cathy uncomfortable. She looked left, right, and up and said to Patricia with a rebuke in her tone, "If you keep on doing what you're doing, how can you have peace?"

Then another patient jumped in. Natalia was a

third aged lady. In the hallways of the clinic, Natalia was the biggest complainer. She took off her glasses and held them in her hand, and said, "Patricia." After a pregnant pause, she continued, "I don't like my situation either. But what can we do? We can take it one day at a time. Since I came here, I saw people worse than me. You know, people like to compare us with others. I don't like that at all." She said louder, "I want to be well. This comparison is not good. I want to be well, and they are telling me that I am better than others, so I should be content." She stopped and took a breath." Humph! We are all struggling daily, and we need to be patient and see how we can deal with that."

"You're right," exclaimed Mrs. Anderson. Mrs. Anderson was probably the oldest in the group. She seemed to be in her late nineties. "I was here sixteen years ago. It was my first stroke, and then I have been here seven more times: another stroke, hip replacement, one thing after another, but I am here in good shape, not in perfect shape, but I am grateful to God for what I have. And let me tell you I am ready to take on more," Mrs. Anderson concluded.

"Patricia," said another patient, with a teary voice. The voice was so teary that it was difficult to hear what she was saying. She shook her head first and continued, "We all want the best, but when we're here, we need somehow to be grateful. At least we have nurses and people who care about us here. I know it is difficult, but we need to celebrate what we have. Don't cry, Patricia. God is watching over us." This statement almost irritated Patricia.

"Do you think that God is watching over us, and we are still here? I don't have that much patience. Where is God, by the way?" She burst into tears and said, "I'm sorry. I shouldn't be saying that."

Almost everyone in the room came to her rescue. "Don't cry, Patricia. Don't cry." They called to her with soft and compassionate voices that seemed to echo in the room.

And Patricia cried louder as the rest of the people moved closer to rescue her. The people in the room forgot about their own situations and focused on Patricia as they tried to comfort her. The chaplain was looking intently. For at least three-quarters of an hour, the conversation between patients brought comfort to each of them.

Patricia stopped crying, and the question became serious. "What should I do?" she asked. "How do you guys cope with this?" It was the beginning of a conversation, each one sharing their story. In the end, it was quiet in the room, with the peace that comes when people really talk things through.

Then the chaplain broke the silence again. "Thank you all for sharing. Your stories and words have been a tremendous gift for each of us. If there are no additional questions or contributions, we can just take prayer requests and pray for each other."

There, through the window, the breeze was shaking the branches of the trees. Sometimes left, sometimes right. The sun had moved to the west and turned the color of the horizon yellow. How did this yellow bowl get there, why, how, when? came to mind. One just wonders what is behind these clouds and this sky.

Maybe the one who listens to the people? Was it listening to us? Was it seeing the tears of people? Did it hear the lyrics, "When the storms of life are raging, Stand by me?" The one people got down on their knees to pray to; the one who saw us "Crying in the chapel, with the tears of joy?" Is it the one who would make our burden lighter;" the one "who never lost a battle?" The one who will give us peace in the valley someday, where there will be no sadness, no sorrow? Where the bear will be gentle, the wolves will be tame, the lion shall lay down by the lamb, and a child will pet the beasts from the wild?"

Maybe these are the songs the trees are playing, moving from one side to another like a philharmonic made only with violin players. But in the room, it was practically the end; the sorrowing faces had given way to faces which are not sad, yet perhaps not smiling, nor hopeful yet. As people continued the discussion between themselves, the turkey had disappeared behind the green leaves, the birds had flown back into the sky, and the deer was nowhere to be found.

This was the beginning of what our other time of prayer and reflection would become. As we started our reflection, we included Packer Palmer in our discussion.

In his book "A Hidden Wholeness, "Packer Palmer addressed the notion of "Deep speaks to deep."

No fixing, no saving, no setting each other straight. Is this the main rule of his reflection? He says that "the shadow behind the fixes we offer for issues that we cannot fix is ironically the desire to hold each other at bay." For Palmer, it is a strategy for abandoning each other while appearing to be concerned. The time of prayer and reflection is not to be used to fix anyone, but it is a time when we learn to listen and speak. We listen to each other, our inner voices, and our own truth and tell our stories.

Our time of prayer and reflection becomes a safe space "for our soul by truthful speaking and respectful listening. We can speak in a particularity powerful form- a form that goes deeper than our opinion, ideas." Palmer agreed that storytelling has always been at the heart of being human because it serves our basic needs—passing along our traditions, confessing, failing, healing wounds, engendering hope, and strengthening our sense of community.

Wood Carven thinks that when we tell our story, we become ourselves. Palmer went in the same direction, saying that we become human when we tell our story. Storytelling allows us to talk to ourselves, listen to our own truth. Truth for Palmer is not "the arrogance of absolutism, "but rather it is 'an eternal conversation' about things that matter, conducted with passion and discipline." When we talk to ourselves, we listen to our own truth. For Palmer, "we speak from our own center to the center of the circle." He made the distinction between types of speech. He spoke about speaking instrumentally and expressively. "When people speak instrumentally, we listen with our own ego, but when people speak expressively, we listen openly with our souls." He explains that "we can attend fully to whatever is being said, knowing that people are not trying to command us and our truth but are making an honest effort to express truths of their own."

Palmer affirmed that we learn to listen to ourselves receptively when we speak in a Circle of Trust. He defines receptive listening as an inward and invisible act. When we listen to others or ourselves, we bring the gift of 'hearing each other into the speech.' Listen brings to us a 'change of heart,' he said. "There are some times when we need to confront scourges. But confrontation often falls short of the transformation. Some people are coerced into short-lived 'change of heart,' while others cling more tightly to the errors of their ways. "This summary of Packer Palmer about 'No fixing- No saving – No setting others straight' brings us to this story.

I recall a story from college. There was a village, far down in the middle of West Africa, near the Sahara Desert. A mission was sent to that area to evaluate the need of the citizens of the village. Early in the morning, while the men were going to the farm, the women took their jars and went out of the town. They came later, at least an hour and a half later, with water. The mission, after four days of observations, concluded that the village needed a well. Their project's main objective was that "a well in the village would help the village people and bring efficiency to their daily activities." So they decided to build the well.

After three months of digging and hard work, the well was finished with the people's help in the village. It was a little celebration; the village people were indeed happy and showed gratitude to the team who made it happen. In a routine patrol, a team member realized that the town's women were not using the well. Every morning, the women were going far to the spring fountain to get some water. It was then that she discovered that it was on their way to the fountain that these women talked about their husbands and many significant things going on in their lives. The report arrived at the university, and many were displeased by the behavior of these women. One of the team members shouted, "I can't believe that it was because of gossip that these women lost all sense of rationality."

We might ask ourselves if it is for gossip or support that these women were travelling to the spring fountain.

These women were living in a community where there was no psychotherapist. The people who were yelling the loudest had access to a psychotherapist when they had a problem. These ladies had their own problems too, so they held their support group while going to the well. It is during these times that they shared their burdens. That probably kept them going and helped them keep their balance. Using the new well would end the spring trip and bring their support group to an end. If that was to happen, their household life might suffer.

The Cartesian rationality is a prominent disease in contemporary academia. Of course, Parker Palmer warned us about fixing, but fixing itself is not the problem. It is the illusion of rationality that people conceive in their heads. In this case, the university mission saw itself as rational. But it is a pure illusion; the village women were rational enough to take the road that will hold their family together and preserve the village life. This is just an example of how irrational we can be if we do not see our rationality as relative.

Rules and regulations

The story of the women and the patients' during the time of prayer and reflection seem totally different. Still, the common ground is to find the "hidden wholeness "in this story. It is, in a different setting, a way of conducting a support group. That way of seeing, of interpreting the women's attitude at the well, opens our eyes to the extreme relativism of pastoral care. The traditional support group is in a room around a table, but here is a support group-taking place on the road. Back to our room, during our time of prayer and reflection, we may consider ourselves on the road, sharing our inner truth. People would share their life stories along this road and leave their burdens at the side of the road before heading to their homes. The road becomes the metaphor for a safe place. The ladies' road to water was a safe place in their community to share their own stories.

The "hidden wholeness" in the attitude of the women of the well symbolizes the preservation of their family. Maintaining their family together is important for the life and the community. The wholeness of that community is hidden in a support group created by the ladies to balance their daily lives. Our role as chaplains is to bring people and help people find their wholeness. To achieve that, we can move from the traditional non-denominational or multi-faith prayer service to a pluri-denominational prayer service.

There is wholeness in every human being. Reflecting and praying can bring people to discover the hidden wholeness in their own lives.

The main rule is to respect each other and affirm the wholeness of our fellow human beings. Our credo is, we celebrate people, respect each other, affirm people in their differences, offer the gift of hearing to each other, and listen to people intently and entirely. The standard non-denominational service implies that we have a language that would not offend anyone. In other words, when we speak in a non-denominational service, our own religion should be hidden so that it might not cause discomfort to our neighbor. This is great and, with no doubt, gives more respect to every one of the people present at the service. The patients in our time of prayer and reflection are in their early stage of disability. Most of them are at the bargaining stage (should I accept this or not?), with deep theodicy questions.

Though their situations are not as they would like, they have a coping skill. These coping skills, good or bad, help the patient somehow during that journey. Coping skills take their source from many aspects of the patients' lives—among them, the emotional and the spiritual. If the spiritual is a part of someone's copying skill, and during the time of prayer and reflection, we refuse to listen to the role of someone's faith in his or her coping skill, then we have not listened to that person totally. It becomes a piece of truth which is not the whole truth. To have someone's "own truth," we need to hear the entire system involved in the coping skill. When we allow people to tell their story and share within their own faith how they came to cope with their situation, we listen to the truth, not a piece of truth. We are affirming that person as a whole. His or her story becomes "their own truth," and listening and affirming people can entirely lead to wholeness and finding the hidden wholeness. During the time of prayer and reflection, the hidden wholeness is that there is wholeness hidden inside every human being. When people share and reflect on their situation, they discover their wholeness through their "own truth-telling."

The leader's role is to set aside that safe place and establish conditions where people can find themselves by listening, speaking, and reflecting.

The pluri-denominational set seems complicated

but doable. The human urgency shows that most human beings tend to worship something. With a simple rule of respect, we can build a community where people are similar in their differences. A pluri-denominational service allows every voice to be heard and brings the unique gift of hearing people sharing their own faith struggle at that time. During our services, the experience we encountered is that most people at that stage of bargaining are not fundamentalist. Most of them question their faith. There are doubts taking place in their minds. The miracle is that when people hear of each other's faith, that they have the same struggles and questions, it brings comfort to say that they are not alone in the journey. The pluri-denominational service affirms and celebrates people. People become one body in their diversity.

The Steps of the Time of Prayer and Reflection:

I- THE LYRICS

The purpose of the lyrics is to prepare people for the reflection. For example, soft songs like Elvis' "Crying in the Chapel," with words that imply self-reflection, help the participants start their own self-examination.

II- THE STORY

We use a popular story. Most people know the purpose of the story is to prevent people from a difficult exercise of their brain or mind. While preventing that exercise, we rather use the popular story to reveal something new. The challenge is that when people can have another view of a story they generally know, they start looking at their own situation in another way. The story should also address the condition of the patient and speak to them directly. In this case, the Ugly Duckling story speaks to the frozen aspects of their life and their own feelings on that journey.

III. THE WISDOM READING

It is generally from a holy book, a word of wisdom from people who have gone through similar trials and tribulations.

IV THE REFLECTION

When there is no objection during the reading, the chaplain's leader can introduce the reflection and let the people continue the reflection. It can be a time for people to share their own truth, story, or viewpoint on any topic in their lives.

V. PRAYER

We ask people to offer prayers or prayer requests loudly or silently, according to their feelings. After all their prayers and prayer requests, the leader can conclude with a general prayer, taking into account all the requests and intentions previously mentioned.

References

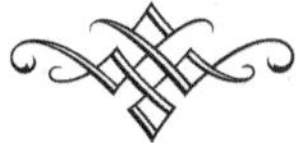

Parker J. Palmer (2009): A Hidden Wholeness, Jossey Bass

Henri J. M Nouwen (1979) The Wounded Healer: Ministry in Contemporary Society

Bill Gaventa (2011) Pastoral Care with Persons with Disabilities and their Families: A Sample Module, Elizabeth Boggs Center, New Brunswick, NJ

Darrell Glenn (1953) Crying in the Chapel, Valley Publishers, Inc., New York.

Hans Christian Andersen, Complete Fairy Tales

John H. Morgan, Clinical Psychotherapy: A History of Theory and Practice (Mishawaka, IN: GTF Books, 2015).

Deirdre Bair, Jung: A Biography (NY: Little, Brown, and Company).

Carl G. Jung, Modern Man in Search of a Soul (NY: Harcourt, Inc., a Harvest Book).

John H. Morgan. Geriatric Logotherapy: Essays in Clinical

Practice and Counseling Psychology. GTF Books (Mishawaka, IN) 2017

John H. Morgan. Clinical Psychotherapy: A History of Theory and Practice. (Mishawaka, IN: GTF Books, 2015).

Sigmund Freud. A General Introduction to Psychoanalysis (Middletown, DE: Renaissance Classic, 2017)

Carl G. Jung, Modern Man in Search of a Soul (NY: Harcourt, Inc., a Harvest Book).

John H. Morgan. Psychopathology: A Clinical Guide to Personality Disorders (South Bend, IN: GTF Books, 2018).

John H. Morgan, Clinical Pastoral Psychotherapy (2012): a practitioner's Handbook for Ministry Professional. 2nd edition, Graduate Theological Foundation, Mishawaka, Indiana,)

Harry Stack Sullivan, Conception of Modern Psychiatry: The First William Alanson White Memorial Lecture, NY: W.W. Norton & Co., 1953.

Viktor Frankl, the Will to Meaning: Foundation and Applications of Logo-therapy, First Meridian Printing (Expanded Edition), New York, Penguin Group, 1988.

Viktor Frankl, Man's Search for Meaning, Boston, Beacon Press 2006.

Parker J. Palmer (2009): A Hidden Wholeness, Jossey Bass

Henri J. M Nouwen (1979) The Wounded Healer: Ministry in Contemporary Society

Bill Gaventa (2011) Pastoral Care with Persons with Disabilities and their Families: A Sample Module, Elizabeth Boggs Center, New Brunswick, NJ

Darrell Glenn (1953) Crying in the Chapel, Valley Publishers,

REFERENCES

Inc., New York.

Hans Christian Andersen (1844) The Ugly Duckling, New Fairy Tales First book, First Collection, C.A. Reitzel, Denmark

Viktor Frankl (1969). The Will to Meaning: Foundation and Application of the Logo-therapy. New York: American Library

Viktor Frankl (1953). "Logos and Existence in Psychotherapy," American Journal of Psychotherapy, VII: 8-15

Viktor Frankl (1961) "Religion and Existential Psychotherapy, "The Gordon Review

Viktor Frankl (1962). "Logotherapy and the Challenge of Suffering, "Pastoral Psychology, XIII

Carl Gustav Jung (1955) Modern Man in Search of a Soul. London: Kegan Paul Trench Trubner, ed (1933)

Carl Gustav Jung. Boligen (1934-1954.) The Archetypes and the Collective Unconscious. (1981 2nd Ed Collected Work Vol. # Part 1) Princeton, NJ.

Viktor Frankl (2004.) An Introduction to Logo-therapy; (Boston; Beacon and Random House/ Rider, London)

Abraham Maslow (1968) Toward a Psychology of Being (2nd Edition)

Carl Rogers. (1961) On Becoming a Person: A therapist's View of Psychotherapy London: Constable.

Peter Gray (1988). Freud: A Life for Our Time (New York: W. W. Norton &Company)

Edward Hoffman (1994). The Drive for Self: Alfred Adler and the Founding of Individual Psychology. (New York: Addison-Wesley Publishing.)

Sigmund Freud (2017). A General Introduction to

Psychoanalysis.

Alfred Adler. (1927) The Practice and Theory of Individual Psychology (1927)

Alfred Adler. (1927) Understanding Human Nature.

Harry Stack Sullivan (1953). Conceptions of Modern Psychiatry: The First William A Alanson White Memorial Lecture, NY: W. W. Norton & Co.)

John H. Morgan (2017). Geriatric Psychotherapy. Essay in Clinical Practice and Counseling Psychology. (Mishawaka, IN: GTF Books , 2015)

John H. Morgan (2014a). Understanding Ourselves: Essays in History and Philosophy of the Social Sciences. (Mishawaka, IN: GTF Books)

John H. Morgan (2015). "Palliative Psychotherapy in the Treatment of Geriatric Depression: A Review of Evidence-Based Psychogenic Options, "Innovative Issues and Approaches in Social Sciences, Vol.8. No1:46-49

Acknowledgment

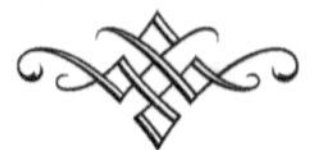

Our gratitude to :

Dr. John H. Morgan

Karl Mannhein Professor of History and Philosophy of the Sciences

Emeritus President and Professor at Graduate Theological Foundation

Senior Fellow at at Foundation House /Oxford

National Science Foundation Fellow at University of Note-Dame

Member of International Advisory Board of the Center for the Study of Religion in Public Life at Kellogg College (Oxford)

Former faculty at Harvard, Yale, Princeton universities .

Rev. William Gaventa

Associate Professor of Pediatric and Director of Community and Congregation support (Ret)at the Elizabeth Boggs Center on Developmental Disability- Robert Wood Johnson Medical School/UMDNJ

Director of Summer Institute on Theology & Disability at Baylor University

Dr. Raynard Smith

Associate Professor of Pastoral Care

Chair of Ministry Studies at New Brunswick Theological Seminary

Rev. Kymberly Clemons-Jones

Pastor of Valley Stream Presbyterian Church

President of Community Caring Center. NY

The faculty at New Brunswick Theological Seminary/ NJ

Kessler Institute of Rehabilitation /NJ

The Graduate Theological Foundation community .

www.ingramcontent.com/pod-product-compliance
Lightning Source LLC
Chambersburg PA
CBHW050847260726
48660CB00006B/2494